STRENGTH BEYOUND FIFTY

Unlocking the Power Within Strategies, Stories, and Secrets for Thriving in Life's Second Act - Navigating Challenges, Embracing Opportunities, and Cultivating Resilience for a Fulfilling and Empowered Life Beyond Fifty

By

Regina P. Wolfe

DISCLAIMER

Copyright © by Regina P. Wolfe 2024.

All rights reserved.

This document may not be replicated or reproduced in any form without permission from the publisher. As a result, the information inside cannot be transferred, stored electronically, or maintained in a database. The publisher or creator must give their consent before any part of the document may be copied, scanned, faxed, or stored.

TABLE OF CONTENT

STRENGTH BEYOUND FIFTY 1

INTRODUCTION 6

CHAPTER 1 8

The Mindset Shift: 8

Adopting a Positive Perspective 8

CHAPTER 2 10

Navigating Physical Health: 10

Strategies for Vitality and Well-being 10

CHAPTER 3 12

Mental Agility: 12

Cultivating Cognitive Resilience and Sharpness 12

CHAPTER 4 15

Embracing Change: 15

Adapting to Transitions and Challenges 15

CHAPTER 5 18

Building Resilience: 18

Overcoming Adversity with Grace 18

CHAPTER 6 21

Relationships and Connection: 21

Nurturing Meaningful Bonds 21

CHAPTER 7 24

Pursuing Passions: 24

Rediscovering Purpose and Joy 24

CHAPTER 8 27

Financial Fitness: 27

Planning for Security and Abundance 27

CHAPTER 9 30

Legacy and Impact: 30

Leaving a Lasting Mark 30

CONCLUSION 33

Tara, a woman of fifty, stood at life's crossroads.

Her children had grown, her career plateaued, and the mirror reflected years of laughter and worry lines etched into her face.

But amidst the uncertainty, a whisper stirred within her:

"There's more to this journey."

Determined to rediscover her spark, **Tara** embarked on a quest of self-exploration.

She embraced challenges with a mix of trepidation and excitement, finding solace in vulnerability and resilience in adversity.

Through reconnecting with old passions and forging new connections, **Tara** unearthed the transformative magic of embracing life beyond fifty.

Each day brought a fresh surge of vitality and purpose. **Tara** savoured the laughter of newfound friends, relished the simplicity of everyday moments, and cherished the wisdom that only comes with age.

Strength beyond fifty isn't just about physical fortitude; it is about embracing life with an unyielding spirit of adventure and a deep-rooted sense of self.

Through **Tara**'s tale, readers are invited on their odyssey of self-discovery, where **empowerment, fulfilment**, and **joy** await in the second half of life.

Beyond the wrinkles and greying hair lies a treasure trove of untapped potential and endless possibilities, waiting to be explored.

INTRODUCTION

Welcome to "**Strength Beyond Fifty**" where we embark on a transformative journey of **resilience**, **renewal**, and **empowerment**. As we proceed into the second half of life, we're met with a landscape brimming with potential and possibility – a terrain ripe for exploration and growth.

In this dynamic space, we'll go deep into the heart of what it means to thrive beyond fifty, transcending societal expectations and limitations to discover our true strength and vitality. Here, age is not a barrier but a gateway to newfound wisdom, resilience, and purpose.

Through captivating stories, insightful reflections, and practical guidance, we'll navigate the complexities of this exhilarating stage of life with courage and grace.

From embracing change and overcoming adversity to cultivating physical well-being and nurturing meaningful connections, we'll uncover the keys to unlocking our full potential and living a life of profound fulfillment.

As we journey through the pages of this book, we'll shatter stereotypes and challenge preconceived notions about aging, redefining what it means to grow older with strength and vitality. Drawing from the wisdom of those who have walked this path before us and the resilience of the human spirit, we'll uncover invaluable insights and practical strategies for navigating life's twists and turns with courage and resilience.

From cultivating a positive mindset and nurturing physical well-being to fostering meaningful connections and leaving a lasting legacy, each chapter will offer a roadmap for thriving in the second half of life.

Along the way, we'll celebrate the victories, embrace the challenges, and discover the hidden treasures that await us in this new chapter.

So, whether you're embarking on this journey with a sense of anticipation or trepidation, know that you're not alone. Together, let's embrace the power of "**Strength Beyond Fifty**" and write the next chapter of our lives with **courage**, **resilience**, and **unwavering determination**.

CHAPTER 1
The Mindset Shift:
Adopting a Positive Perspective

"**The Mindset Shift**: Adopting a Positive Perspective" is not merely a change in thought patterns; it's a profound shift in the very essence of how we perceive ourselves and the world around us.

It's about embracing the idea that our mindset shapes our reality, and by choosing to see the world through a lens of positivity, we can transform our experiences and well-being.

Essentially, adopting a positive outlook involves nurturing a mindset characterized by appreciation and strength. It entails recognizing the obstacles and difficulties that aging may bring, while deliberately directing our attention towards the wealth of blessings and possibilities that remain in our future.

It's about transforming setbacks into opportunities for personal development and enlightenment, rather than allowing them to hinder our sense of contentment.

This mindset shift requires a willingness to let go of old beliefs and societal expectations about aging.

It invites us to embrace our journey with open arms, recognizing the inherent value and wisdom that come with each passing year. It encourages us to cultivate self-compassion and kindness, both towards ourselves and others, as we navigate the ups and downs of life.

Practical exercises and actionable strategies serve as tools on this journey, helping us to cultivate **resilience**, **foster optimism**, and find **joy** in the present moment.

Through reflection and introspection, we uncover the power of our thoughts and beliefs to shape our reality, and we harness this power to create a life filled with **purpose**, **meaning**, and **fulfillment**.

In essence, "**The Mindset Shift**: Adopting a Positive Perspective" is an invitation to embrace the fullness of life with gratitude, resilience, and unwavering optimism.

It's a reminder that no matter our age or circumstances, we have the power to choose how we perceive and experience the world, and by choosing positivity, we unlock the door to a future filled with limitless possibilities.

CHAPTER 2

Navigating Physical Health: Strategies for Vitality and Well-being

Navigating Physical Health: Strategies for Vitality and Well-being embarks on a journey toward holistic wellness, recognizing that our physical health is the cornerstone upon which our overall well-being is built.

In this chapter, we explore not only the importance of maintaining physical health as we age but also practical strategies for doing so in a way that fosters vitality, resilience, and longevity.

Managing physical well-being involves adopting a lifestyle that harmonizes with our body's inherent rhythms and requirements.

This entails consuming nutritious foods, staying adequately hydrated, and participating in enjoyable physical activities regularly. However, it extends beyond mere fundamentals; it involves attuning to our body's cues, respecting them, and according to them the care and consideration they merit.

We delve into the importance of movement, not just as a means of staying fit, but as a way to connect with our bodies and enhance our overall well-being. From gentle exercises like yoga and tai chi to more vigorous activities like hiking and swimming, we explore the myriad ways in which movement can invigorate our bodies, sharpen our minds, and nourish our souls.

Through **mindfulness**, **meditation**, and other **relaxation techniques**, we cultivate a sense of balance and harmony that supports our **physical**, **emotional**, and **spiritual well-being**.

Managing physical health transcends the pursuit of flawlessness or rigid adherence to strict guidelines; rather, it revolves around embracing a lifestyle that respects the individual requirements of our bodies and promotes vitality throughout every phase of life.

By prioritizing self-care, attuning to our body's signals, and approaching health with an attitude of curiosity and kindness, we establish the groundwork for a life brimming with vigor, resilience, and vibrant well-being.

CHAPTER 3

Mental Agility:

Cultivating Cognitive Resilience and Sharpness

Mental Agility: Cultivating Cognitive Resilience and Sharpness embarks on a route into the intricate workings of the mind, recognizing that our cognitive health is just as vital as our physical well-being.

We would explore the importance of maintaining mental agility as we age and delve into practical strategies for sharpening our minds and cultivating resilience in the face of life's challenges.

At its core, mental agility is about fostering flexibility, adaptability, and creativity in our thinking. It's about challenging ourselves to learn new skills, explore new ideas, and embrace new perspectives, even as we navigate the complexities of life.

By engaging our minds in stimulating activities and exercises, we can enhance our cognitive abilities, improve our memory and concentration, and protect against cognitive decline.

From reading and writing to engaging in puzzles, games, and other mental exercises, exploring myriad ways in which one can keep our minds sharp and engaged.

In addition to cognitive exercises, exploring the role of **mindfulness** and **meditation** in promoting mental clarity and resilience. By cultivating present-moment awareness and practicing non-judgmental acceptance, we can train our minds to respond more effectively to **stress**, **uncertainty**, and **adversity**.

Cultivating cognitive resilience and sharpness is not about staving off the effects of aging or achieving perfection; it's about embracing the fullness of our cognitive abilities and nurturing them with care and intention.

By adopting a growth mindset, staying intellectually curious, and approaching challenges with flexibility and creativity, we can navigate life's twists and turns with clarity, confidence, and resilience.

Moreover, mental agility involves nurturing emotional intelligence and resilience, recognizing that our thoughts and feelings are deeply intertwined. By cultivating self-awareness, self-regulation, and empathy, we can navigate life's ups and downs with greater ease and grace.

Through mindfulness practices and emotional intelligence exercises, we learn to manage stress, regulate our emotions, and cultivate a sense of inner peace and balance.

In today's fast-paced world, where information overload and constant distractions abound, it's more important than ever to cultivate cognitive resilience and sharpness. We explore strategies for managing digital overwhelm, such as setting boundaries with technology, practicing digital detoxes, and engaging in activities that promote focus and concentration.

Furthermore, we delve into the importance of brain-boosting nutrition and lifestyle habits, recognizing that what we eat and how we live can profoundly impact our cognitive health.

So it's very vital that by fueling our bodies with nutrient-rich foods, staying physically active, and prioritizing sleep and relaxation, we can optimize our brain function and protect against cognitive decline.

CHAPTER 4
Embracing Change:
Adapting to Transitions and Challenges

Embracing Change: Adapting to Transitions and Challenges invites us on a profound journey through the ever-shifting landscapes of life. It's a journey marked by uncertainty, yet illuminated by the promise of growth, resilience, and newfound possibilities.

At its core, embracing change is about acknowledging the inevitability of life's transitions and choosing to greet them with open arms, rather than shrinking away in fear.

In this chapter, we embark on a heartfelt exploration of the diverse forms change takes in our lives – from the subtle shifts of our daily routines to the monumental transformations that reshape our paths.

Through personal anecdotes, collective experiences, and pragmatic guidance, we'll navigate these transitions with grace and fortitude, discovering resilience in adversity and embracing newfound opportunities amidst the tumult of change.

One of the most profound benefits of embracing change is the opportunity for personal growth and self-discovery. When we step outside of our comfort zones and embrace new experiences, we open ourselves up to a world of possibilities.

We learn more about ourselves – our strengths, our weaknesses, and our true desires – and we become more resilient, adaptable, and open-minded in the process.

Moreover, embracing change allows us to break free from the constraints of the past and step into a future filled with unlimited potential. By letting go of outdated beliefs, habits, and patterns of behavior, we create space for new opportunities to emerge.

We become more **creative**, **innovative**, and **resourceful** in finding solutions to life's challenges, and we develop a sense of empowerment and agency over our destinies.

But embracing change isn't always easy – it requires courage, resilience, and a willingness to face uncertainty head-on. There are practical strategies we can employ to navigate life's transitions with greater ease and grace.

Mindfulness practices, such as meditation and deep breathing, can help us stay grounded and present amidst the chaos of change. Self-care rituals, such as exercise, journaling, and spending time in nature, can nourish our bodies, minds, and spirits, giving us the strength and resilience we need to weather life's storms.

Embracing change is a choice – a choice to let go of the past and step into a future filled with endless possibilities. It's a choice to greet life's transitions with **curiosity**, **courage**, and an **open heart**, knowing that each change, no matter how challenging, is an opportunity for growth, transformation, and self-discovery.

So let's embrace change with open arms, knowing that on the other side lies a brighter, more fulfilling future waiting to be discovered.

CHAPTER 5
Building Resilience:
Overcoming Adversity with Grace

Building Resilience: Overcoming Adversity with Grace invites us to embark on a deeply personal journey of inner strength and fortitude.

It's a journey marked by the inevitable trials and tribulations of life, yet illuminated by the unwavering belief in our ability to rise above them with grace and resilience.

Essentially, constructing resilience involves nurturing the internal capacities necessary to confront life's obstacles with bravery, perseverance, and resilience.

It entails acknowledging that adversity is an unavoidable aspect of being human, yet refusing to allow it to dictate our identity. Instead, adversity can catalyze personal development, metamorphosis, and the discovery of newfound fortitude.

One of the most profound benefits of building resilience is the ability to bounce back from setbacks stronger and more resilient than before. When we cultivate resilience, we develop the skills and mindset needed to overcome obstacles with grace and dignity. We become more adaptable, flexible, and resourceful in the face of adversity, and we develop a deep sense of inner strength and confidence that carries us through life's toughest challenges.

Moreover, building resilience allows us to find meaning and purpose amid adversity. When we face setbacks, we have the opportunity to learn from them, grow from them, and ultimately, use them as stepping stones to a brighter future.

We discover our inner resilience and capacity for growth, and we find solace in the knowledge that even in our darkest moments, there is light to be found.

But building resilience isn't always easy – it requires dedication, commitment, and a willingness to face our fears head-on. Fortunately, there are practical strategies we can employ to cultivate resilience and overcome adversity with grace.

Mindfulness practices, such as meditation and deep breathing, can help us stay grounded and present amidst the chaos of life's challenges. Self-care rituals, such as exercise, journaling, and spending time with loved ones, can nourish our bodies, minds, and spirits, giving us the strength and resilience we need to weather life's storms.

Constructing resilience is a voyage – an expedition of self-exploration, expansion, and metamorphosis. It demands that we welcome our vulnerabilities, confront our fears, and transcend our constraints with courage and poise.

Ultimately, this journey propels us toward a realm of inner **fortitude**, **resilience**, and **steadfast confidence** in our capacity to surmount any obstacle that life presents.

Let us eagerly embrace the endeavor of cultivating resilience, fully aware that on the horizon awaits a future imbued with brightness and fortified resilience, yearning to be uncovered.

CHAPTER 6
Relationships and Connection: Nurturing Meaningful Bonds

Relationships and Connection: Nurturing Meaningful Bonds is an invitation to embark on a journey of human connection and profound intimacy. It transcends the superficial and delves deep into the heart of what it means to truly connect with others in a meaningful and authentic way.

Fostering meaningful connections involves cultivating bonds that enhance our existence, infusing it with happiness, satisfaction, and a profound feeling of belonging.

It entails acknowledging the intrinsic significance of human relationships and purposefully dedicating ourselves to nurturing those that hold the greatest importance in our lives.

One of the most profound benefits of nurturing meaningful bonds is the sense of connection and belonging it brings into our lives.

When we invest in nurturing our relationships, we create a support network of friends, family, and loved ones who stand by us through life's ups and downs.

We feel **seen**, **heard**, and **understood**, and we know that no matter what challenges we may face, we are not alone.

Additionally, nurturing meaningful bonds enables us to relish the joy of shared experiences and cherished memories.

Whether it involves sharing laughter with friends over a cup of coffee, engaging in heartfelt conversations with loved ones, or simply basking in the presence of cherished companions, these instances of connection serve as poignant reminders of life's inherent beauty and profound richness.

But nurturing meaningful bonds isn't always easy – it requires time, effort, and a willingness to be vulnerable. It means showing up authentically, listening with an open heart, and being willing to extend grace and forgiveness when needed.

It means prioritizing connection over perfection and being willing to invest in the messy, imperfect, yet deeply rewarding work of building relationships.

Fortunately, there are practical strategies we can employ to nurture meaningful bonds and cultivate deeper connections with others.

Simple acts of kindness, such as expressing gratitude, offering support, and showing empathy, can go a long way in strengthening our relationships and deepening our connections. Regular communication, whether through **phone calls**, **texts**, or **face-to-face interactions**, helps to keep our relationships alive and thriving, even amid life's busyness.

In the grand scheme of things, nurturing meaningful bonds is a heartfelt odyssey – one that demands our full presence, openness, and vulnerability with ourselves and those we hold dear.

It's a transformative journey that leads us to a deeper comprehension of ourselves and those around us, paving the way for a life imbued with richness, fulfillment, and a profound sense of love, connection, and belonging.

Let us wholeheartedly embrace the endeavor of nurturing meaningful bonds, knowing that beyond lies a realm of boundless potential and profound connection, waiting to be explored.

CHAPTER 7
Pursuing Passions:
Rediscovering Purpose and Joy

Pursuing Passions: Rediscovering Purpose and Joy is an exhilarating exploration of the soul's deepest desires and the transformative power of following our heart's calling.

This beckons us to rediscover the spark of inspiration within us and to reignite the flames of purpose and joy that fuel our lives.

At its essence, pursuing passions is about honoring the unique **gifts**, **talents**, and **interests** that make us who we are. It's about listening to the whispers of our soul and daring to dream big dreams, no matter how impossible they may seem.

It's about reclaiming our sense of agency and autonomy, and boldly charting a course toward a future filled with meaning, fulfillment, and boundless possibility.

One of the most profound benefits of pursuing passions is the sense of purpose and fulfillment it brings into our lives.

When we engage in activities that light us up and bring us joy, we tap into a wellspring of **creativity**, **inspiration**, and **vitality**.

We feel alive, energized, and fully present in the moment, and we experience a deep sense of satisfaction knowing that we are living authentically and in alignment with our true selves.

Moreover, pursuing passions allows us to cultivate a deeper connection with ourselves and the world around us. Whether it's through creative expression, physical activity, or intellectual pursuits, engaging in activities that we love helps us to tap into our inner wisdom and intuition, and experience a profound sense of flow and ease.

We lose track of time, and our worries and cares melt away as we immerse ourselves fully in the present moment.

But pursuing passions isn't always easy – it requires courage, perseverance, and a willingness to step outside of our comfort zones.

It means facing our fears and insecurities head-on, and daring to believe in ourselves and our dreams, even when the odds are stacked against us.

It means being willing to embrace failure as a natural part of the creative process, and to use setbacks as opportunities for growth and learning.

Fortunately, there are practical strategies we can employ to pursue our passions and rediscover purpose and joy in our lives. Setting aside dedicated time for activities that bring us joy, surrounding ourselves with supportive friends and mentors, and cultivating a growth mindset are just a few of the ways we can nurture our passions and create a life filled with purpose and fulfillment.

Finally, pursuing passions is a journey of self-discovery and self-expression – a journey that invites us to reclaim our power and live life on our terms.

It's a journey that leads to a deeper understanding of ourselves and the world around us and to a life filled with meaning, fulfillment, and boundless joy.

So let's embrace the challenge of pursuing passions with open hearts and open minds, knowing that on the other side lies a world of infinite possibility and limitless potential.

CHAPTER 8
Financial Fitness:
Planning for Security and Abundance

Financial Fitness: Planning for Security and Abundance is a transformative expedition into the realm of financial well-being, where we learn to harness the power of planning, discipline, and abundance mindset to cultivate a life of security and prosperity.

Financial fitness is not just about accumulating wealth; it's about building a foundation of stability and freedom that empowers us to live life on our terms.

It's about taking control of our finances, rather than letting them control us, and creating a future filled with security, abundance, and peace of mind.

One of the most profound benefits of achieving financial fitness is the sense of security and peace of mind it brings into our lives. When we have a clear plan for our finances and a solid financial foundation to fall back on, we can weather life's storms with confidence and resilience. We feel empowered to take risks, pursue our passions, and live life to the fullest, knowing that we have the resources and support we need to thrive.

Moreover, achieving financial fitness allows us to cultivate a mindset of abundance and prosperity. Instead of living in fear and scarcity, constantly worrying about making ends meet, we embrace a mindset of abundance, believing that there is more than enough to go around and that we are worthy of experiencing financial success and prosperity.

This abundance mindset opens us up to new opportunities and possibilities and allows us to attract wealth and abundance into our lives with ease and grace.

But achieving financial fitness isn't always easy – it requires dedication, discipline, and a willingness to make tough choices and sacrifices in the short term for long-term gain.

It means living within our means, avoiding unnecessary debt, and making smart financial decisions that align with our values and goals. It also means being willing to seek out help and guidance when needed, whether through financial advisors, mentors, or support groups.

There are practical strategies we can employ to achieve financial fitness and create a life of security and abundance.

From creating a budget and sticking to it to paying off debt and building an emergency fund, to investing wisely for the future, there are steps we can take to take control of our finances and create a brighter, more prosperous future for ourselves and our loved ones.

Achieving financial fitness is a journey – a journey of self-discovery, discipline, and empowerment. It's a journey that requires us to take control of our finances and create a future filled with security, abundance, and peace of mind.

So let's embrace the challenge of achieving financial fitness with open hearts and open minds, knowing that on the other side lies a life of **security**, **abundance**, and **unlimited potential**.

CHAPTER 9
Legacy and Impact:
Leaving a Lasting Mark

Legacy and Impact: Leaving a Lasting Mark is an exploration of our innate desire to create a meaningful imprint on the world and the profound ripple effects of our actions.

It's a journey that transcends the bounds of time, inviting us to reflect on the legacy we wish to leave behind and the impact we aspire to make on future generations.

At its essence, legacy and impact are about more than just material wealth or personal achievements; they're about the lasting impression we leave on the lives of others and the world around us. It's about the values we uphold, the relationships we nurture, and the contributions we make to the greater good.

One of the most profound benefits of embracing the idea of legacy and impact is the sense of purpose and fulfillment it brings into our lives. When we align our actions with our values and work towards a cause greater than ourselves, we tap into a deep wellspring of meaning and significance. We feel connected to something larger than ourselves, and we derive a sense of joy and satisfaction knowing that our efforts are making a positive difference in the world.

Moreover, embracing the idea of legacy and impact allows us to cultivate a sense of gratitude and humility, recognizing that we are part of a larger tapestry of human experience. We acknowledge the contributions of those who came before us and the role we play in shaping the future for generations to come.

This sense of interconnectedness inspires us to live with intention and purpose, and to leave behind a legacy that reflects our deepest values and aspirations.

But embracing the idea of legacy and impact isn't always easy – it requires **courage**, **resilience**, and a **willingness** to step outside of our comfort zones. It means confronting our fears and insecurities, and daring to dream big dreams, even when the odds are stacked against us.

It means being willing to take risks and embrace failure as a natural part of the journey towards making a meaningful impact.

There are practical strategies we can employ to cultivate a legacy of impact and leave a lasting mark on the world.

From volunteering our time and resources to supporting causes that align with our values, to mentoring and inspiring others to reach their full potential, there are countless ways we can make a positive difference in the world around us.

Embracing the idea of legacy and impact is a journey – a journey of self-discovery, growth, and transformation. It's a journey that invites us to reflect on what matters most to us and to live our lives with intention and purpose.

So let's embrace the challenge of leaving a lasting mark with open hearts and open minds, knowing that on the other side lies a world of infinite possibility and boundless potential.

CONCLUSION

The journey through "**Strength Beyond Fifty**" explores the depths of the range of human experience. Every chapter offers priceless insights and practical solutions for overcoming life's obstacles with **bravery, elegance**, and **unwavering determination**.

These strategies range from accepting change and building resilience to developing meaningful connections and following personal passions.

We are reminded of our intrinsic power to control our fates as we reflect on the recurrent themes woven throughout this journey: from mental adjustments to accepting uncertainty, from building resilience to making a lasting impression.

It is shown that growing older does not have to be a barrier, but rather a doorway to new possibilities.

We have explored the depths of the human spirit and discovered the **resiliency, bravery**, and **boundless potential** inside each of us via poignant stories, group experiences, and practical advice.

When we accept the challenges that come our way, we grow into more **resilient**, **intelligent**, and **compassionate people** who are better able to overcome any roadblocks.

Let us take with us the lessons learned from these pages as we navigate the paths of life: the importance of embracing change, the fortitude exhibited in the face of difficulty, and the enormous impact of cultivating meaningful relationships and pursuing personal passions.

May we bravely, tenaciously, and with unflinching faith in our ability to thrive, whatever the obstacles we face, steadfastly embrace the "**Strength Beyond Fifty**" adventure.

And may we never forget the innate fortitude and resiliency that every one of us possesses, leading us toward a future full of abundance, joy, and meaning.

www.ingramcontent.com/pod-product-compliance
Lightning Source LLC
Chambersburg PA
CBHW070957220526
45471CB00007B/3073